The Littlest Daffodil

For Ella,
the bravest daffodil I know

Written by Lele Ste
Illustrations by Kathy Peterson

First edition: August 2015

ISBN-13: 978-1517153984
ISBN-10: 1517153980

Printed in the United States of America

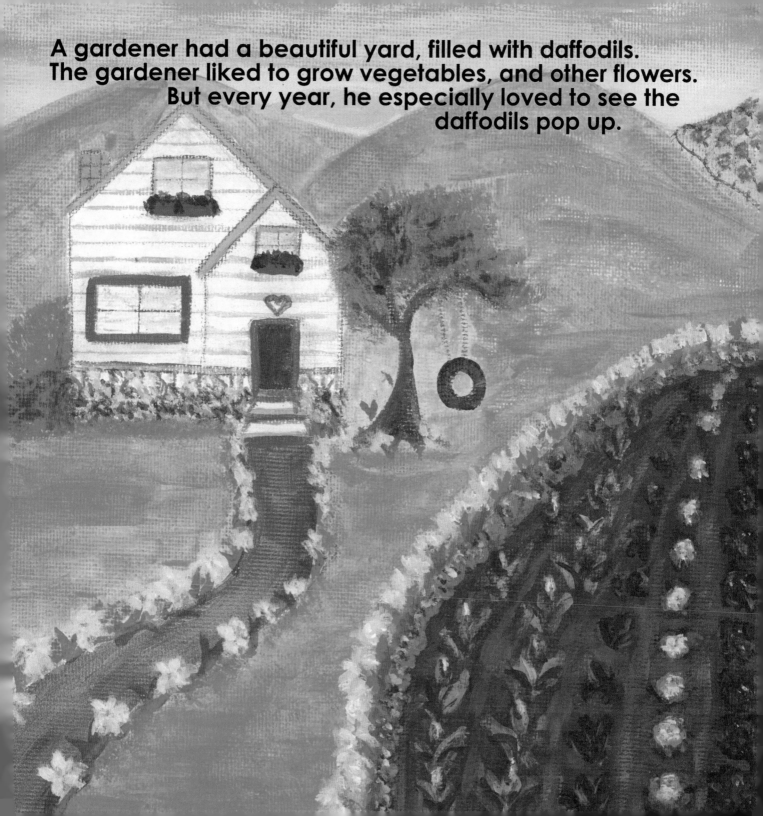

A gardener had a beautiful yard, filled with daffodils.
The gardener liked to grow vegetables, and other flowers.
But every year, he especially loved to see the
daffodils pop up.

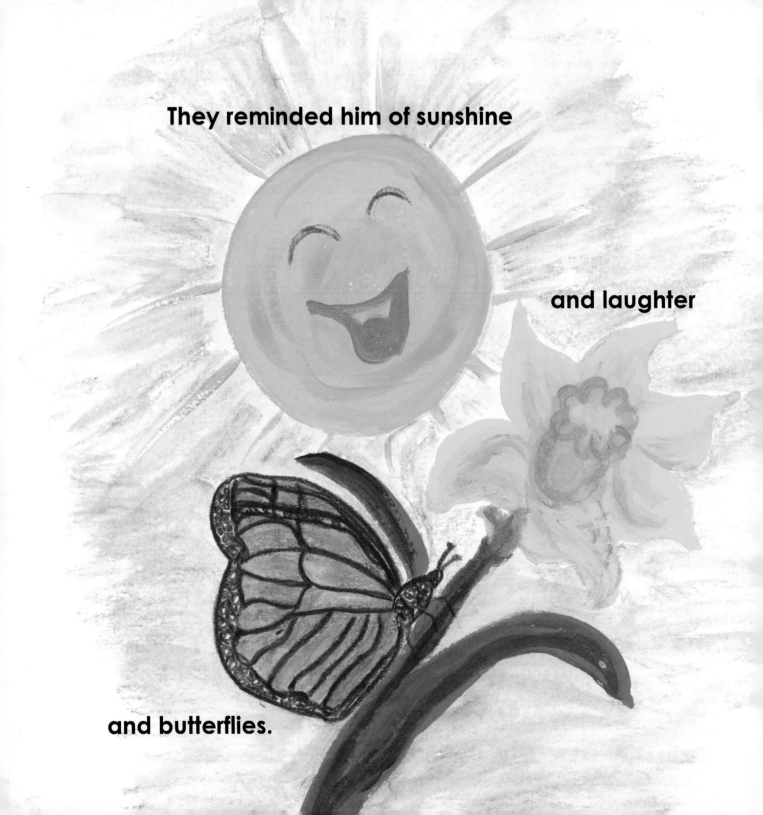

They reminded him of sunshine

and laughter

and butterflies.

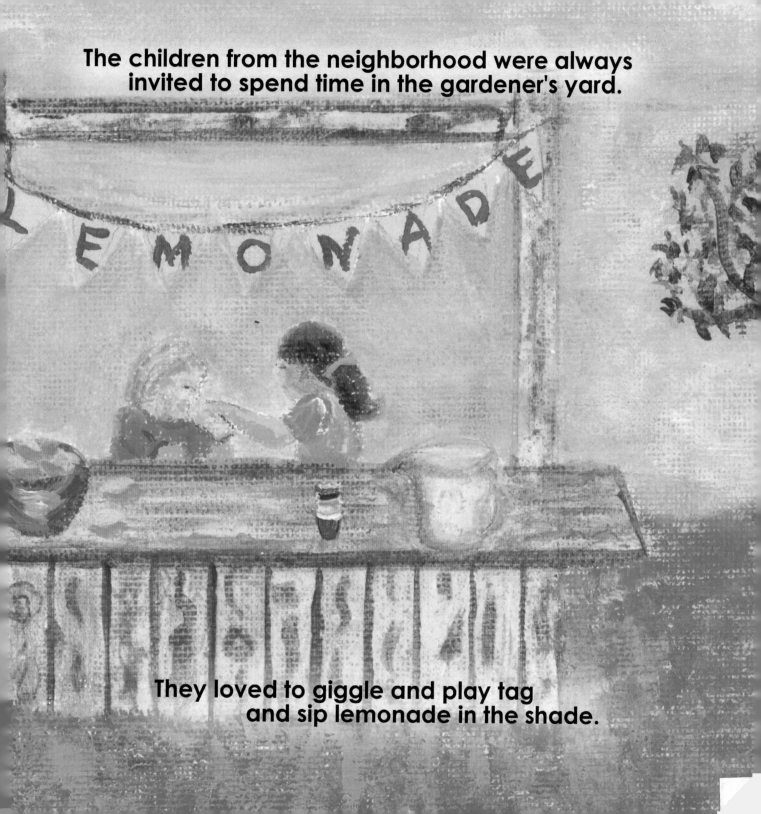

The children from the neighborhood were always invited to spend time in the gardener's yard.

They loved to giggle and play tag and sip lemonade in the shade.

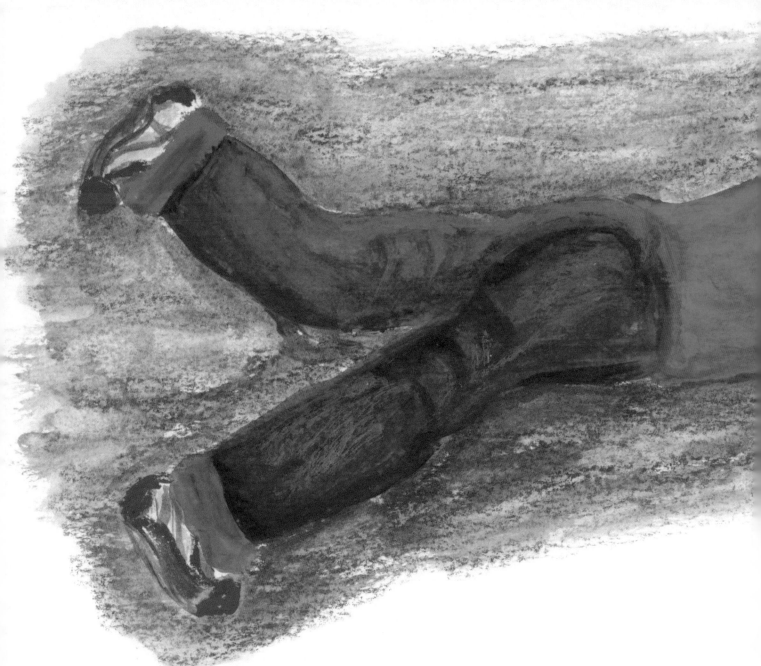

**One day, when the children were playing
and laughing with their cups of tasty lemonade,
a little boy ran too close to the daffodils.**

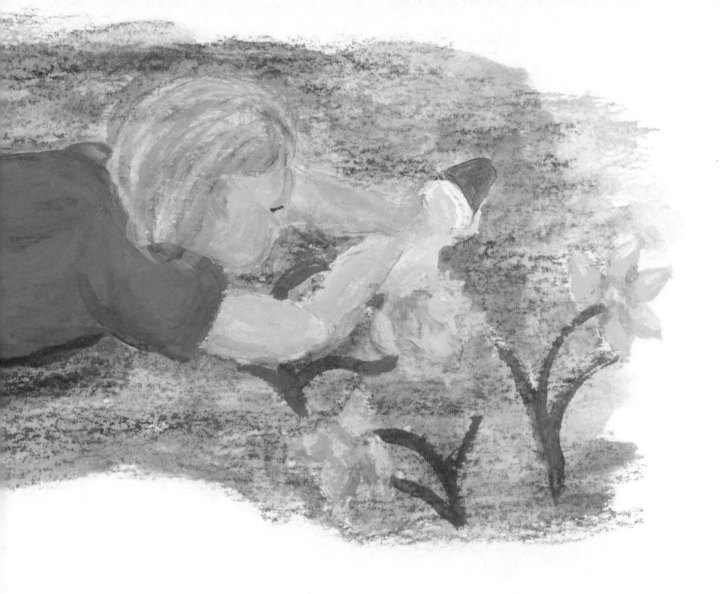

"Watch out!" said the gardener, but it was too late.
The boy fell right on top of the little daffodil,
spilling his lemonade all over the small flower.

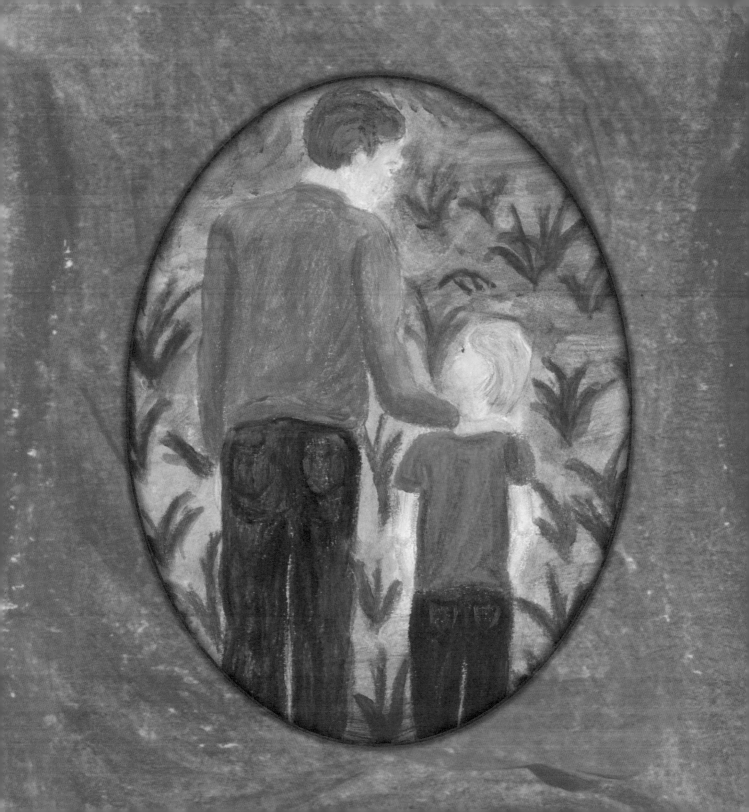

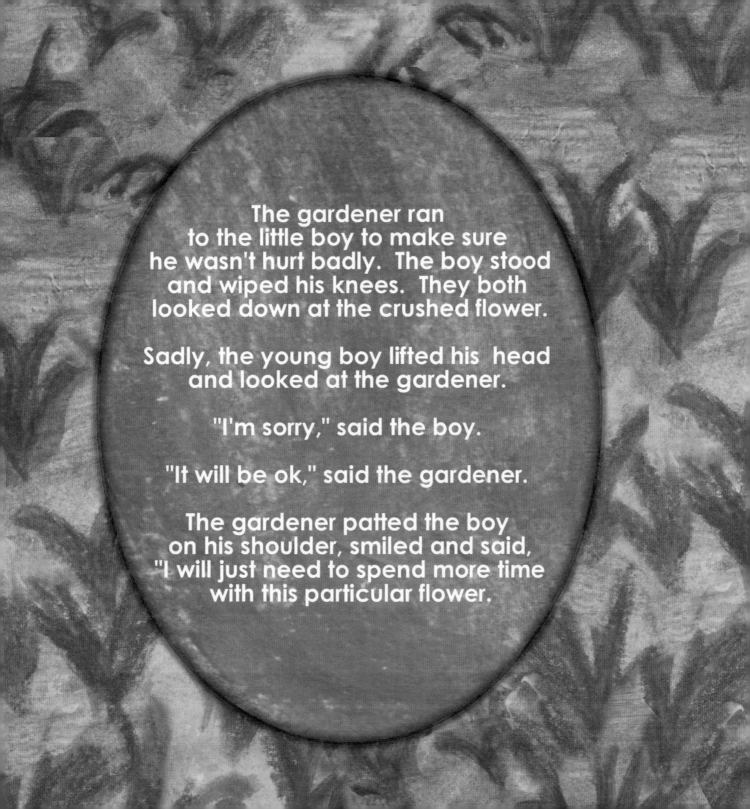

The gardener ran
to the little boy to make sure
he wasn't hurt badly. The boy stood
and wiped his knees. They both
looked down at the crushed flower.

Sadly, the young boy lifted his head
and looked at the gardener.

"I'm sorry," said the boy.

"It will be ok," said the gardener.

The gardener patted the boy
on his shoulder, smiled and said,
"I will just need to spend more time
with this particular flower.

That night, the daffodil cried and cried.

The other daffodils couldn't make her feel any better.

She hurt all over.

One of the closest flowers leaned over in the evening breeze
and whispered gently to her.

"It will be alright, little one.
The gardener will take good care of you."

But the daffodil was very scared, and she cried and cried
until she finally fell asleep very late in the evening.

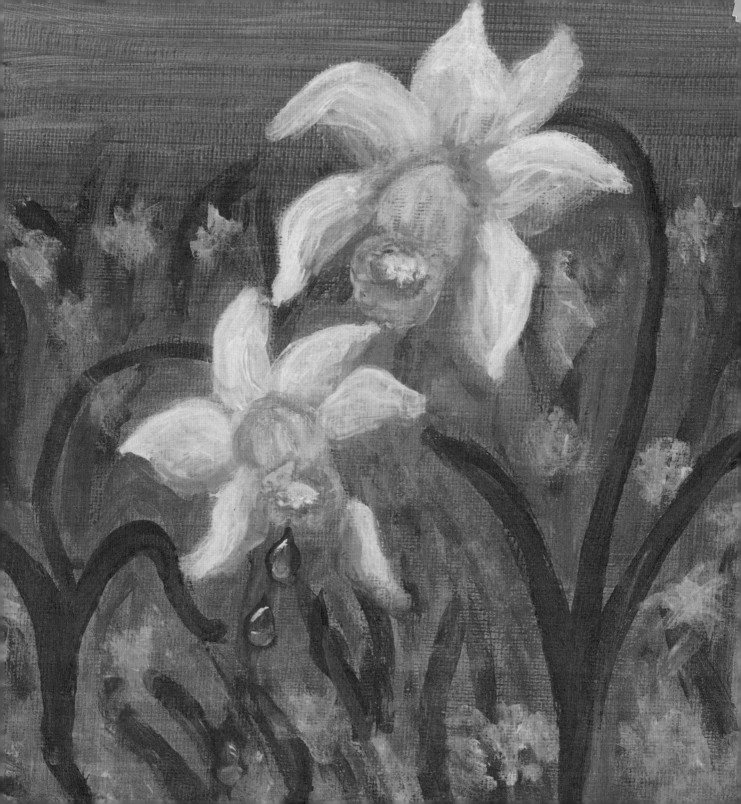

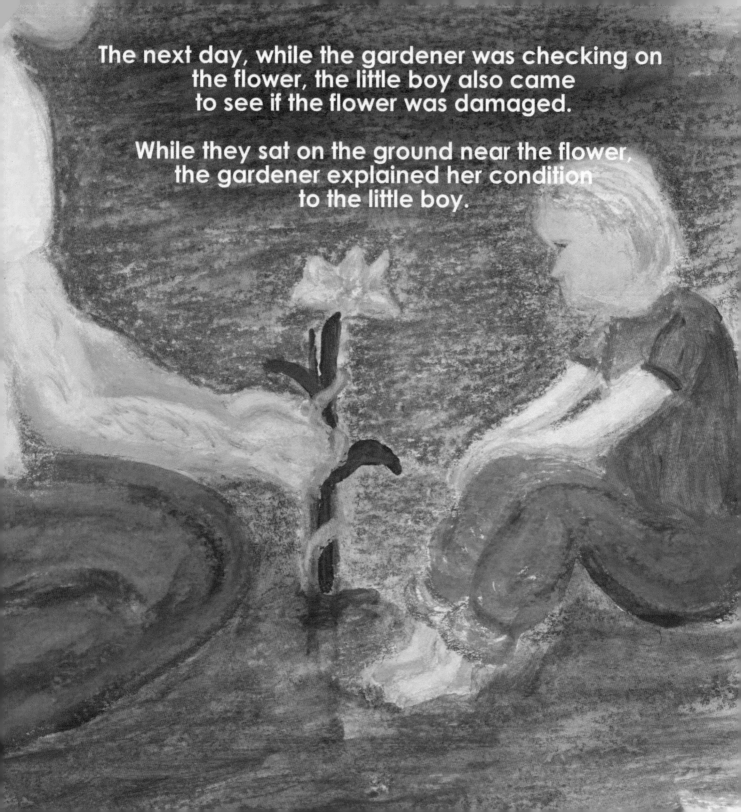

The next day, while the gardener was checking on
the flower, the little boy also came
to see if the flower was damaged.

While they sat on the ground near the flower,
the gardener explained her condition
to the little boy.

"Her stem was bruised," said the gardener, "and her petals are very fragile right now, but her roots are strong."

As the little boy watched, the gardener gently wrapped twine around two sticks placed near her stem.

"This will help her stem to grow strong again."

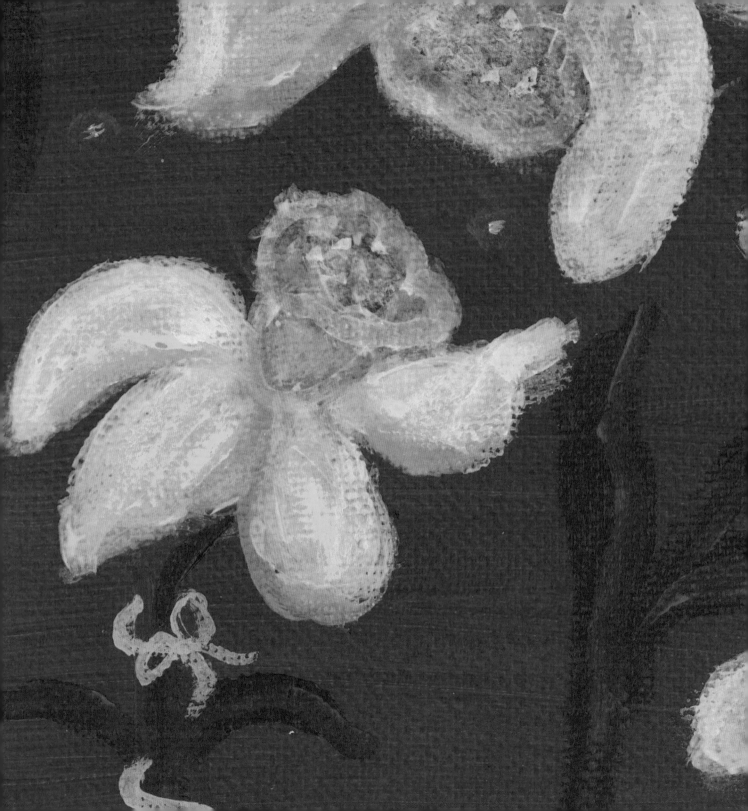

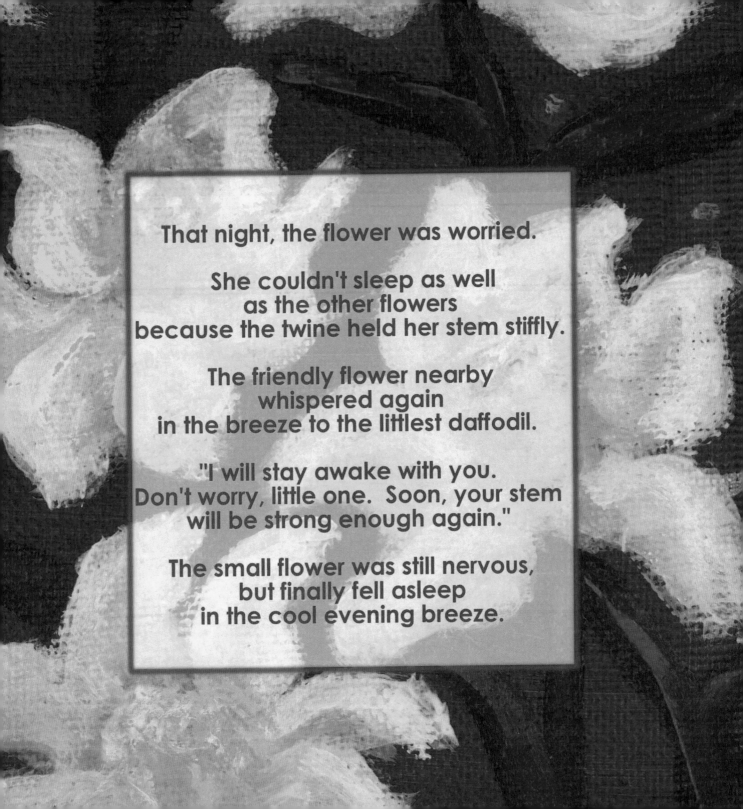

That night, the flower was worried.

She couldn't sleep as well
as the other flowers
because the twine held her stem stiffly.

The friendly flower nearby
whispered again
in the breeze to the littlest daffodil.

"I will stay awake with you.
Don't worry, little one. Soon, your stem
will be strong enough again."

The small flower was still nervous,
but finally fell asleep
in the cool evening breeze.

The next day, while the gardener tended the flower,
the little boy came again.

Do you see how green her
leaves are? That's good!

She needs her leaves to make
food, but see this?

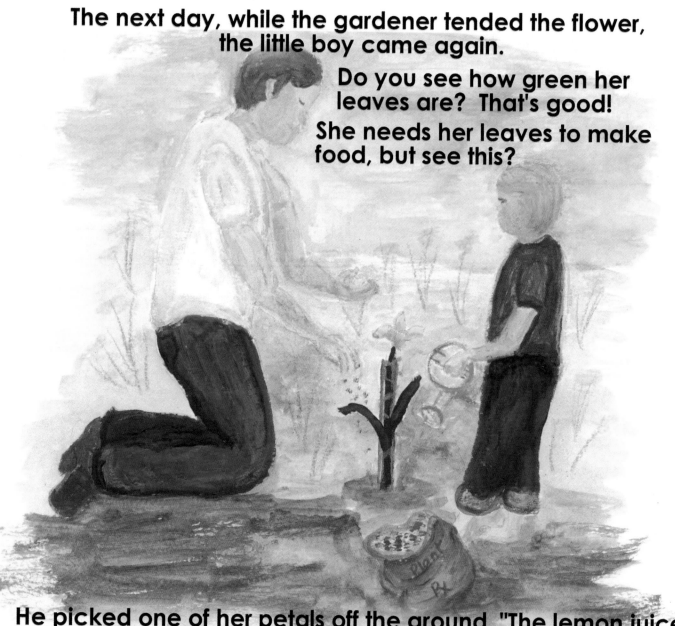

He picked one of her petals off the ground. "The lemon juice
from the lemonade went into her soil and did some damage.
We will need to add water and extra nutrients to the soil
around this flower." As he added the medicine to the the soil,
he hummed a beautiful song over the flower.

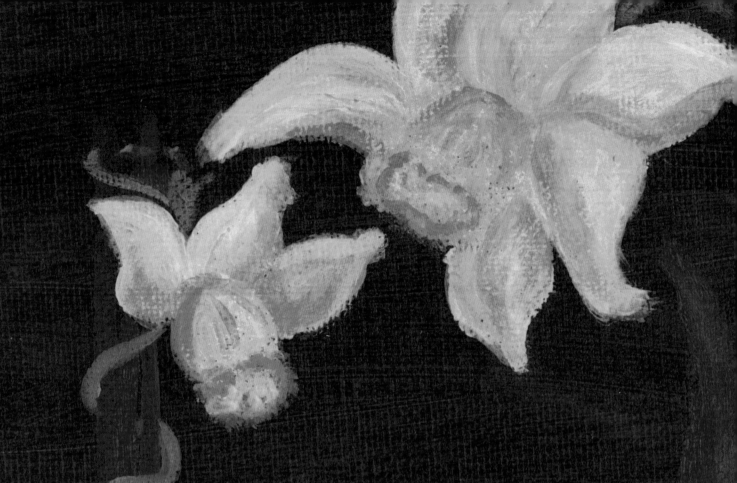

That night, the little flower looked at the other flowers.
They had all their petals. She could feel her missing petal.
She didn't like that.

The nearby flower bent to her in the evening breeze.
"Don't worry, little one. Your stem is getting stronger
and your leaves are nice and green.
Petals are nice, but they aren't necessary."

The little daffodil didn't want to sleep. She only stared sadly
at the hundreds of other daffodils with all of their petals.

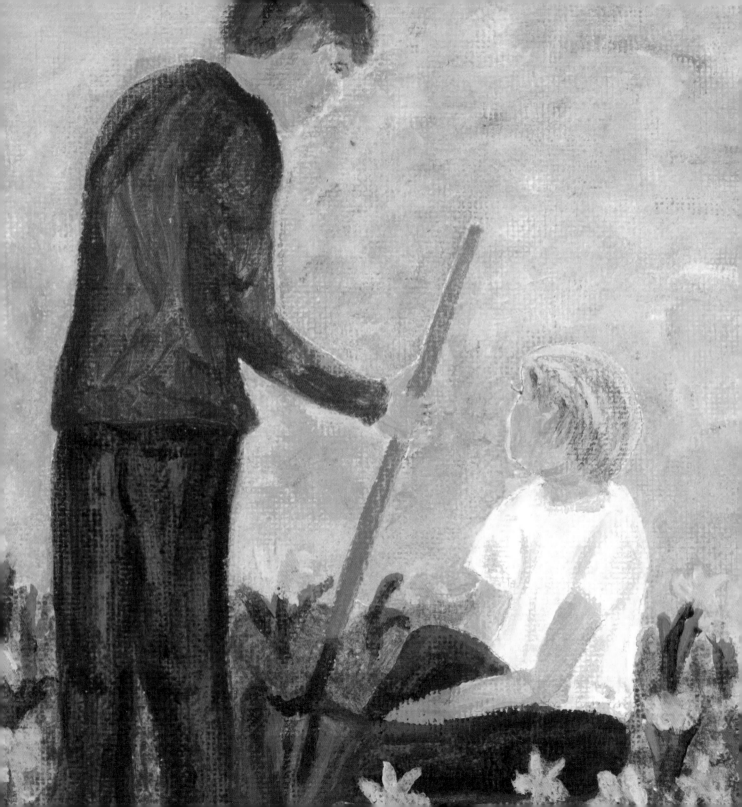

The next day, while the gardener tended the flower, the little boy sat very close to the daffodil. They both gently picked up all of the petals that had fallen in the night.

The little boy looked at the daffodil. It didn't look like all of the other flowers. He looked to the gardener and asked quietly, "Do you have to throw that daffodil away now?"

"Oh no!" said the gardener. "This daffodil has become one of my very special and very favorite flowers in all of my garden. I have spent so much time caring for this little one. I have enjoyed humming to her while I carefully pour water into her soil.

I smile when I see how strong her stem has become, because of my caring touch.
Just wait and see. We hold her petals in our hands now, but next year when she grows, I think she will grow stronger and more beautiful than ever before!"

The little boy thought about that, but then looked at all the other flowers around her. "But she looks so different than all the other daffodils," said the boy.

The gardener looked around too, and nodded his head. "Yes, you're right. She is different. She is unique! When I look at her, I see how beautiful and strong she is. I think about how much time we have spent together. I love how she looks."

That night, even though the little daffodil had no petals, she looked around at all the other flowers and she was glad for all the special time she had spent with the gardener. The nearby flower bent over to her in the evening breeze.

"How do you feel, little one?"

The little daffodil answered,
"I feel unique, and special.
I feel beautiful and strong.
The gardener said that I am all of those things,
and I believe him!"

And as she started to fall into sweet sleep,
she hummed the special song the gardener had sung to her.

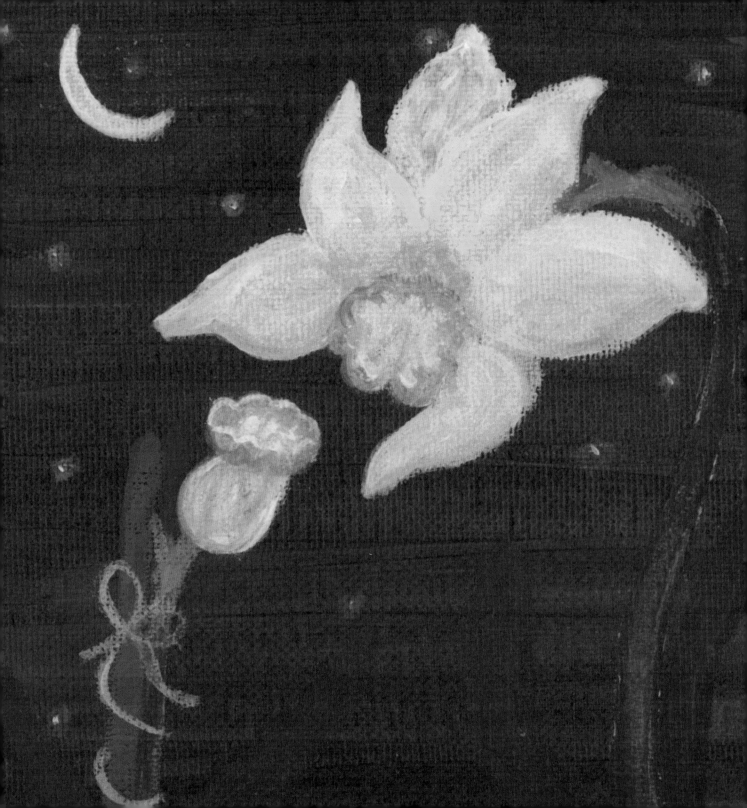

The next year, the little boy came to see the daffodils.
He smiled a big smile as he found the little daffodil.

It was just as the gardener said.
She was more beautiful than ever before.

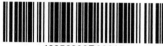

Made in the USA
Charleston, SC
15 November 2015